HAPPY JOINTS

the yoga
for
arthritis
handbook

HAPPY JOINTS: The Yoga for Arthritis Handbook

by: Kim McNeil
layout and design by: Lawrence Zalasky
cover illustration by: Janice Blaine
photography by: Voyager Photography
additional photography by: Noah Fallis

Find Kim on the web at: **www.kimmcneilyoga.ca**

First Printing
Printed in Canada
ISBN: 978 - 0 - 9921448 - 0 - 7

This book is dedicated to Pat, Chris, and my beautiful friend Sof, all of whom live with arthritis. They taught me to never take a move for granted.

To my clients and students with arthritis, and to all of you. May you find inner ninja strength to karate chop arthritis so you can feel better and live happier.

Thank you

To all those who shared their stories with me, thank you for helping to inspire this book.

Rebecca Garland, who inspired me with her own book and showed me it can be done. You pushed me to stay accountable to myself, to keep it simple, and to not let setbacks get in the way of a good thing.

Mellisha Fehr, for showing me that you can be a fierce business women but still keep your soul. Thank you for guiding me to look for the signs...and for being my partner in crime.

Susi Hately, for her guru yoga business guidance. Thank you for teaching me the importance of finding my own voice. It is because of you that I learned the significance of putting my work on paper to share with others.

Janice Blaine, for her beautiful artwork that was the seed from which the book grew.

My clients and students, who practiced the sequences and gave me honest feedback. You make me a better teacher every day.

Margot Kitchen, the most magical teacher I have ever had. Thank you for molding me into the teacher I am today.

Baldur the dog, my pooch who taught me what is important in life. He was never far away when I was writing, practicing the sequences, or in need of a break to go for a walk.

Lawrence Zalasky, my husband and ridiculously talented graphic designer. I never wanted anyone else to get their hands on this project. This book is beautiful because of your professional eye, style, and passion for the work. I could not have done it without you. Thank you for believing in me and for your laughter along the way. Elephant shoe.

Health is a state of complete harmony of the body, mind and spirit. When one is free from physical disabilities and mental distractions, the gates of the soul open.

~ B.K.S. Iyengar

contents

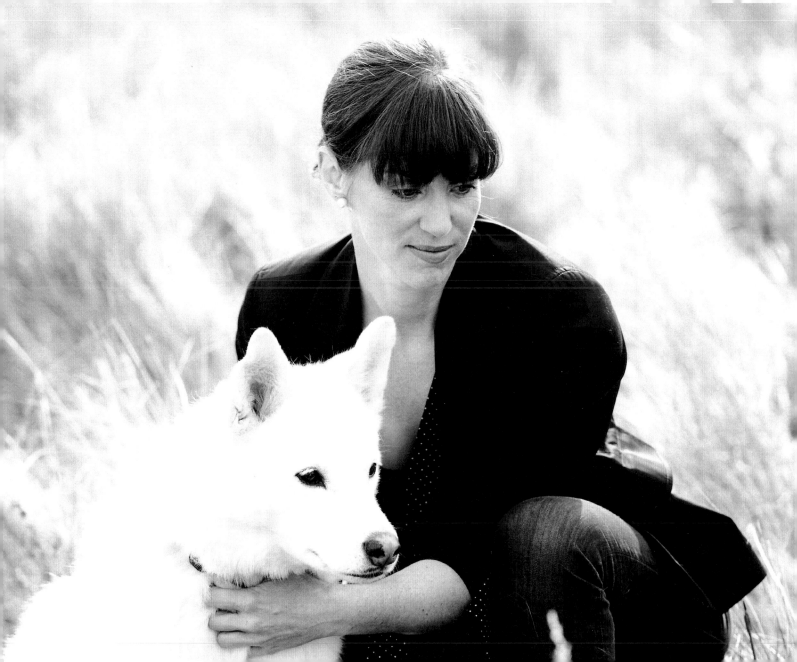

the story

I had heard too many stories about how arthritis had reduced the quality of life of my family, friends, and students. Their stories were eerily similar: they went undiagnosed for years, they felt older than their age, and they had given up doing the things they loved to do. Many felt frustrated that others didn't "get it" when it came to understanding what they were going through. They felt controlled by their arthritis and planned their days around avoiding embarrassment or pain. When it came to exercise, they felt there were not enough options that catered to their needs.

I knew yoga could help with the pain, stiffness, stress, and even depression that goes along with arthritis. I had heard the testimonials from complete strangers about how my yoga had helped them feel human again. I saw the changes that were made in my client's bodies. I decided there should be a resource just for them, something they could use at home every day that empowered them to take control of their lives and feel better again.

I hope this book does what I had hoped it would: help those living with arthritis feel better and, ultimately, live a happier life.

Here's to happy joints,

how to use this book

First off, buy the book. If you can't buy it, steal it.

Read over the part on '**Fundamentals**'. Read it out loud. Write it down. Tell a friend. Do whatever it takes to memorize it. There's no quiz at the end but learning the '**Fundamentals**' is the key to you getting the most out of this book and your new yoga practice.

Turn to the part of the book that discusses the area or areas of the body that speak to you. For example, if you experience hip pain or your hips are tight, head to:

The Lower Body: Hips

Each chapter gives you a sequence of modified yoga ninja moves to help you conquer your problem areas. Follow the principles of practicing for each and every sequence.

The sub-sections titled '**Evolution**' were created for those who have reached 'Ninja Master' status to allow you to progress to the next level. Here I give you variations, and sometimes full poses, that build upon on basics. Don't skip the foundational stuff though! Often the simple poses are the most challenging, both physically and mentally.

Who This Book Was Made For

This book was made for you if:

- you live with **arthritis**.
- you feel older than your age.
- one of your goals is to **get back to doing the things you love to do**, like knitting, karate, or space travel.
- you were diagnosed 1 month ago or 40 years ago and are between the ages of 0 and whatever age you are.
- you want to learn how to add yoga to your toolset to **manage your pain and other symptoms**.
- you are a **wanna-be yoga ninja** who wants to empower themselves instead of always relying on someone else.
- **you are a teacher** who wants to learn how to better serve your students living with arthritis.
- **you are a cheerleader for someone with arthritis** and you are trying to better understand their needs.

What to Expect

The Handbook will teach you:

- how to **break down yoga poses into smaller parts** so that you can enjoy improved range of motion, better joint function and less pain.
- how to **modify traditional yoga poses** for your body.
- which poses will give you the **biggest bang for your buck** depending on where you feel symptoms.
- **how to use breathing** to help manage pain, reduce stress, and build your body awareness.
- **the importance of keeping your joints** mobile within their safe, natural range of motion.
- **how to pace yourself** using yoga to gain more strength, flexibility, and mobility.
- **why meditation is cool** and not just for hippie tree hugging yogis.
- how to be a **yoga ninja.**

fundamentals

As you work through this book, remember the **Ten 'Happy Rules' or Fundamentals** for a safe yoga practice. These guidelines are based on exercise physiology, yoga therapy, physiology and anatomy, body mechanics, results from my private practice, and plain old personal experience.

1. Think holistically

Your body is not a hodgepodge of independent parts but rather a collection of brilliantly designed pieces that make up a larger puzzle (the 3D kind). Each joint, muscle, tendon and ligament is intimately connected to several others. For example, stop thinking of "the knee" as a stand alone piece, instead think of it as part of a multi-joint chain.

Expand this idea to your other various parts; poses for the shoulders can also help the hips; poses for the foot can help the back. I've designed 'The Handbook' with this idea in mind: **think of your body as a whole and approach your yoga practice as something that cares for all of it.**

2. Range of motion: quality over quantity

When it comes to **movement**, we often think more is better. We speed through moves without really feeling and we force joints into places they shouldn't go. We also push past our safe limits and we ignore warning signs - increased pain, clicking in joints, compensation, muscle strain, holding our breath. Less is more when moving your joints. Aim for quality of movement over quantity and **move only what you need to**. For example, when you lift your arms overhead, are you forced to arch your back or zigzag your arms into position?

Listen to your body; move to your safe and comfortable range but not past and slowly progress from there. You will create new neuromuscular patterns to retrain your body to move safely and more effectively, use the correct muscles, and with less, or even no, pain.

- Move slowly and mindfully
- Move without pain (or without increasing pain)
- Work only what you need
- Learn your limits

3. Think strength, not flexibility

Tight muscles are often weak. It doesn't make sense to approach a therapy-based yoga practice from the standpoint of stretching only. When we think of yoga as stretching, it can backfire on us by creating the exact opposite result we were looking for: a further tightening of a muscle group instead of the development of more flexible muscles.

Muscles can be tight from underuse, from overuse or from protecting and stabilizing arthritic joints. Having strong, resilient muscles willing to let go when they should will do wonders for maintaining good joint health.

Use, don't abuse, your muscles.

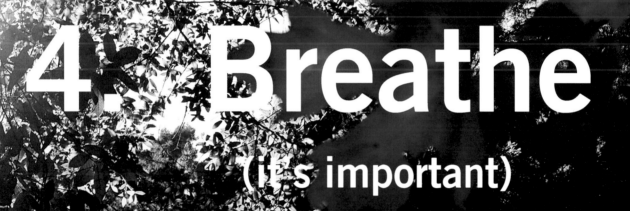

4. Breathe

(it's important)

5. Move, move, move

When you have arthritis and pain, your instinct may be to protect or avoid using your joints. It might seem obvious coming from a yoga book, but to be clear: **you must move your joints to keep them healthy.**

6. Look for elephants

It can be confusing at times to decide what to work on in your yoga practice. When you have arthritis, you want to tackle everything that ails you. You could have multiple joints that hurt as the pain migrates week to week or month to month. But there is only so many hours in the day to dedicate to your practice. My tip: focus on the areas that speak to you. Are there areas in the body where, from the right side of the body to the left, you feel the biggest difference in strength, flexibility, and/or mobility? If so, focus your time and energy there. Look for the differences or the elephants in your body.

7. R&R: Care for your psychological and physical health.
(physical and emotional integration)

The holistic approach goes beyond our physical parts. Stress plays a role in how we manage pain and the pain and anxiety caused by arthritis often leads to depression. This book will help you build body awareness, ninja-like mental strength, and the ability to focus on your breathing, three of your biggest allies when it comes to managing pain.

Once you are ready to fight arthritis with your newly acquired ninja skills, it can be tempting to go full steam ahead with your practice. Remember to schedule in rest days to give yourself a mental and physical break.

Take care of all of you to help conquer stress and you will feel better.

8. Start each day with a fresh perspective

The difference between a yoga practice and simply going through the motions of a therapy program is that yoga teaches us that every day is different. Every time you hit the mat the experience and your perspective will be new. This is refreshing because it gives us the opportunity to let go of pre-conceived ideas about how our practice should be or how we will feel day-to-day. Take the idea of svadhyaya, the study of oneself and one of the 5 niyamas of yoga, with you every time you practice. Accept what your body can and can not do on any given day. Use your tapas or discipline to continue your practice even when you would rather crawl out of your own skin.

9. Learn acceptance

Pain sucks but it can also be an useful warning sign to tell us when something is up. The difficulty with this rule of thumb is that when we have arthritis we are often in pain. Our bodies are programmed to want to avoid any discomfort. What ends up happening is we find ourselves in a constant fight with our own bodies. Learn to accept your body and your arthritis and you will feel better, happier, and be in less pain. Practice ahimsa or friendliness when it comes to loving the body you have; learn santosha or contentment to find ways to be happy in every moment.

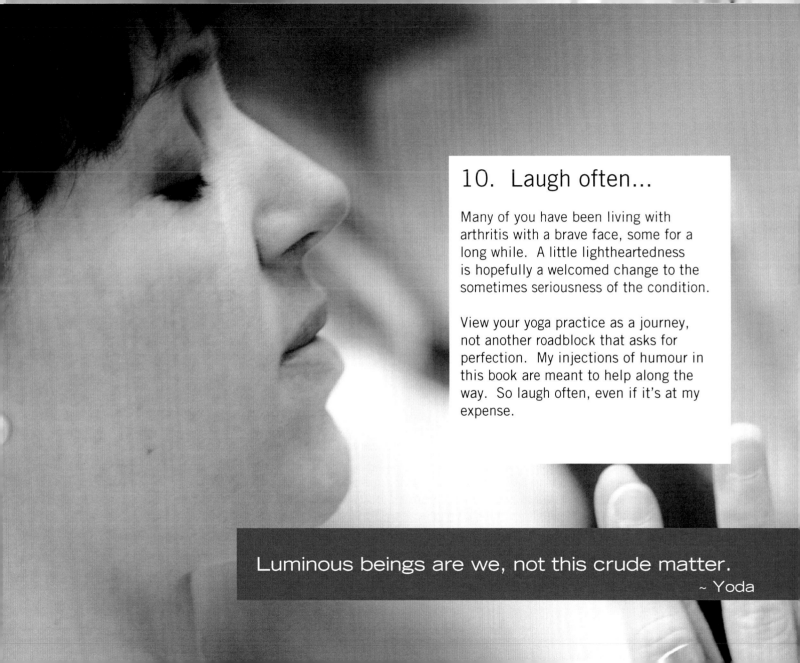

10. Laugh often...

Many of you have been living with arthritis with a brave face, some for a long while. A little lightheartedness is hopefully a welcomed change to the sometimes seriousness of the condition.

View your yoga practice as a journey, not another roadblock that asks for perfection. My injections of humour in this book are meant to help along the way. So laugh often, even if it's at my expense.

Luminous beings are we, not this crude matter.

~ Yoda

Joints

Joints are where two bones meet, they hold your skeleton together and allow you to move. Most of your joints are designed to move which is why immobility is one of the greatest threats to joint health. In order to understand why, you first need to understand a little bit of joint physiology...

Types of Joints

There are three types of joints in your body: Fibrous, Cartilaginous, and Synovial.

Fibrous or Fixed joints don't allow for any movement and are held together by fibrous connective tissue. The joints of your skull are fixed joints.

Cartilaginous or Semi-movable joints, like those between vertebrae of the spine, allow for some movement. A gelatinous but firm substance called cartilage cushions and connects the bones that make up these joints.

Synovial joints are the most flexible and common type of joint in your body; they make up the joints of your limbs. Ligaments stabilize these joints while muscles move them. The Handbook will focus mainly on these joints

Joint Shape

The shape of joints gives you a clue about how they function. Once you know their shape, you can better understand how they should and should not move.

Ball and socket joints are the most mobile type of joint in your body. Both the hip and shoulder joints are ball and socket joints. An example of a movement created by a ball and socket joint is the hip rotation in Tree Pose or Vrksasana, or a Ninjutsu kick.

Hinge joints create movement around a fixed point. Your fingers, knees and elbows are examples of hinge joints. An example of a hinge joint movement is the bent knee in Warrior I or Virabhadrasana I, or a Ninjutsu arm chop.

Pivot joints allow rotation. For example, the pivot joint in your neck allows you to turn your head from side to side, and the shape of the bones in your forearm allow you to rotate your forearm for a Ninjutsu death punch.

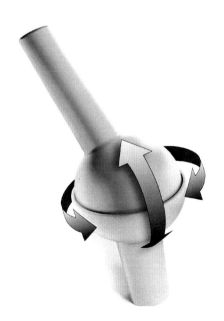
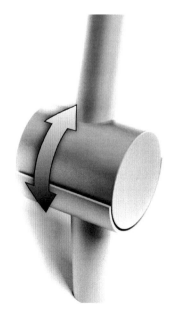
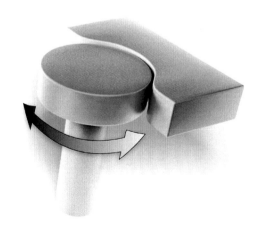

Joint Structure

Synovial joints have the cushioning articular cartilage of semi-movable joints but with an added layer of lubricating liquid called synovial fluid. Think of it like motor oil for your joints. This fluid is contained within a joint capsule which protects, supports, and nourishes the joint.

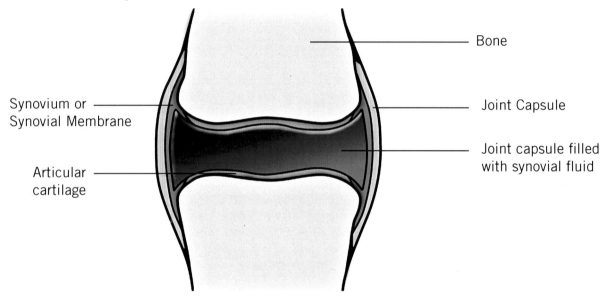

Bone

Joint Capsule

Joint capsule filled with synovial fluid

Synovium or Synovial Membrane

Articular cartilage

The capsule is lined with layers of cells which make up the synovial membrane called the synovium. These cells are what produce the lubricating synovial fluid which carries oxygen, protein, glucose, and other goodies to the joint. The fluid also acts as shock absorber, friction reducer, and supplier of nutrients to the cartilage. Don't let the figure fool you: the fluid-filled space between the bone cartilage surfaces is very thin.

Still with me? Hang in there...

Joint cartilage and synovial fluid have a close relationship. The porous cartilage is like a sponge: when it is squeezed, it releases fluid; when it expands, it draws up fluid. By doing this, joint cartilage releases metabolic waste and absorbs nutrients to and from the fluid. The fluid is constantly being replaced so it can continue to do its job. While at rest, the exchange of synovial fluid by the spongy cartilage is slow, but when you move the exchange speeds up.

The articular cartilage that covers the joint surfaces allow for the bones that make up the joint to glide easily along one another. However, the cartilage is fragile and susceptible to damage. The result can be arthritis.

In some joints like the knee, the cartilage is helped by the meniscus, a rubbery fibrocartilage substance. When a joint undergoes pressure, the meniscus is there to help provide structural support, distribute applied forces, and increase the overall function of the joint.

Joint Movement

Joints wouldn't budge without the help of ligaments, muscles, and tendons. Bones are held together at joints by ligaments. These fibrous connective tissues help to stabilize joints by properly aligning bones.

Muscles attach to bones at joints by tendons. Muscle contractions are what cause joints to move and apply forces to bone which in turn help to build and maintain bone strength.

Cue yoga.

Yoga, Joint Health, and Arthritis

During an uber cool yoga for arthritis class, the contortions of the poses promote the circulation of fluid as the cartilage and the joint capsule flex and expand. The best part is when joints are moved into their full healthy range of motion, fluid is moved around the entire inside of the joint coating cartilage in the nutrient rich fluid.

There's a tiny catch: push yourself past your healthy range and you risk injuring not only your muscles, ligaments, and tendons but also your joint capsules. Learn your limits and listen to your body to keep your joints happy.

The take-home message: yoga, yoga, yoga. I mean movement. **Your joints need to move to stay healthy!**

the lower body

The Feet and Ankles

Rock n' Roll your feet - Self-myofascial Release

It's a little uncomfortable, but don't let that scare you; the benefits to your body awareness, fascia, and flexibility are well worth the brief discomfort.

Prop: Tennis ball or Spiky ball

Tip: If you are new to this technique, opt for a tennis ball and then a golf ball before advancing to the spiky ball of dread.

How to: Roll out your bare feet using the spikey ball from either a seated or standing position, whichever is more comfortable and accessible to you.

- Roll back and forth across the foot starting from the heel and moving your way up to the ball of the foot.
- Change directions, rolling up and down your foot.
- Roll in a circular motion to finish off.
- When you feel a 'hot spot', one where there is greater sensitivity, stop rolling and allow your foot to melt over the ball.
- Go to your happy place, breathe, and feel what happens.
- Explore one foot for ~ 2 minutes; switch feet.

Legs Up the Wall - Viparita Karani

Prop: Wall, blanket (optional)

How to: Lay on your back with your legs supported against a wall. Place a thinly folded blanket under your back for support if you feel discomfort along your spine. Adjust your distance from the wall so the backs of your legs feel comfortable (no stretch in your hamstrings) and your buttocks remain on the floor. Bend your knees slightly if needed. Your spine and pelvis should stay neutral and in contact with the floor throughout.

Tip: Knees and thighs should remain still, no bending or rotating, throughout the pose.

Heel Press:

- **Neutral:** Inhale and press up gently through the center of your heels using the muscles of your shins, exhale to release. As you press your toes should stay level as if they were making a shelf. **Repeat for 10 breaths.**

- **Outer-heel (inversion):** Repeat as above but press the outer edges of your feet up. Your outer toe mounds will press up so that your feet angle outer-edge up. **Repeat for 10 breaths.**

- **Inner-heel (eversion):** Repeat as above only this time press the inner edge of your feet up. Your inner toe mounds will press up so that your your feet angle inner-edge up. **Repeat for 10 breaths.**

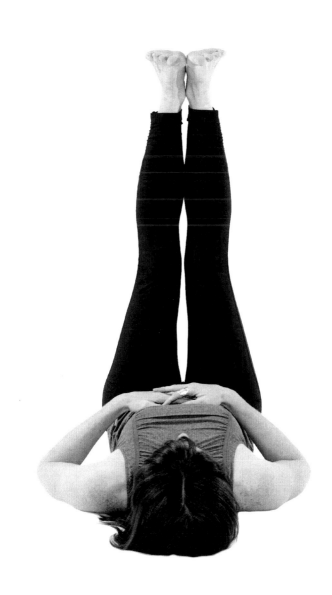

Like a Bird: Pigeon - Penguin

Tip: Move slowly with with ease to respect your range of motion and to avoid knee pain.

- Move your legs into a small "V" about hip width apart.

- Pigeon (adduction): Move like a pigeon. Turn your feet in so your forefeet move towards the midline of the body. **Repeat for 10 breaths.**

- Penguin (abduction): Get in touch with your inner penguin. Turn your feet out so your forefeet move away from the midline. **Repeat for 10 breaths.**

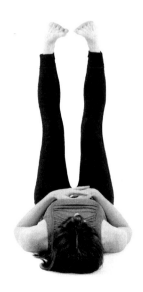 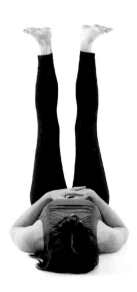

Mountain Pose - Tadasana

How to: Stand with your feet shoulder-width apart, equal weight on both feet. Ground evenly through the three points of the feet: heel, outer edge and big toe mound. Roll your shoulders back as you relax your arms at your sides. Look straight ahead as you focus on one spot. Engage your thigh and buttock muscles to help keep your legs strong and your pelvis neutral.

Tip: Move from your ankles, not from your knees, hips or spine. Don't allow yourself to bend at hips or arch your back as you sway.

Tip: Keep the three points of your foot grounded throughout

Ankle Sways (Balance) - To practice pronation and supination and to improve ankle mobility:

- Stand in Tadasana.

- Slowly shift your weight forward, like a ski jumper, and backward. **Move with your breath and repeat for 10 breaths.**

- Now sway from side to side. **Move with your breath and repeat for 10 breaths.**

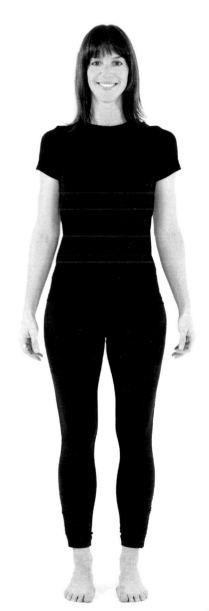

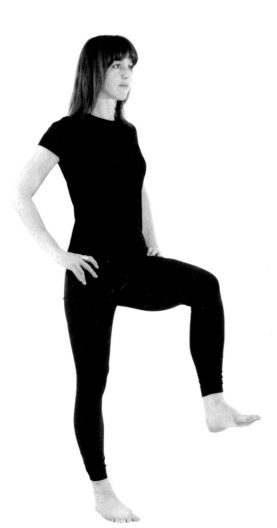

Shins - 2 Ways

Prop: Wall or chair, or for a more advanced variation, practice this as a balance pose.

Tip: Your thigh should stay still throughout. Be especially picky when you do the shin rotations that the movement comes from your knee, not your hip.

- Stand in Tadasana next to a wall or a chair to help with balance.

- Shift your weight to your left foot and lift your right foot off the floor as you bend your right knee. Your knee should be no higher than hip height.

- **Ankle flex:** Inhale and bend (dorsiflex) your right ankle, exhale to release. Use the muscles of your shin to pull your right foot up while you keep the toes relaxed. **Repeat for 10 breaths or less if that's all you can muster, then switch legs.** Move with the breath.

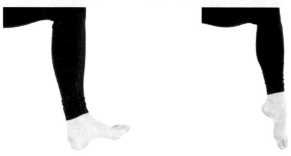

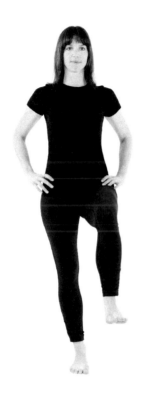 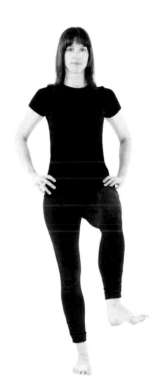

- **Shin rotation**: Inhale and rotate your right shin out to the right, exhale to return to center. Keep your toes relaxed and your kneecap pointed forward. **Repeat for 10 breaths or less then switch legs**.

The Knees

Leg Lifts

Prop: Floor or a bed

How to: Lay on your back on the floor or on a bed. Bend both knees then straighten one leg out along the floor, this will be the leg you will lift. Start by engaging your thigh muscles and lift your entire leg from the floor, hold for a breath, then lower. **Repeat for 10 breaths then switch legs.**

Tip: Imagine someone pulling up on a string attached to the centre of your thigh to lift your leg. If you feel the muscles of the front of the hip engage as you lift the leg, you have lifted the leg too high. A good rule of thumb is lift no higher than 30°.

- **Neutral leg:** The straight leg should have the knee cap and toes pointing up to the ceiling. Inhale and lift your leg, exhale to release.
- **External rotation:** Rotate the straight leg out. Inhale and lift the leg as if the string was attached to your inner thigh, exhale to release.
- **Internal rotation:** Rotate the straight leg in. Inhale and lift the leg as if the string was attached to your outer thigh, exhale to release.

Tip: If you practice one of the rotated leg options, make certain it is the thigh bone that is rotating in the hip socket, not the shin or ankle turning.

Evolution #1: Supta Padangustasana - Practice with your lifted heel resting against a wall, pillar or door frame. Gently pull your leg away from the wall.

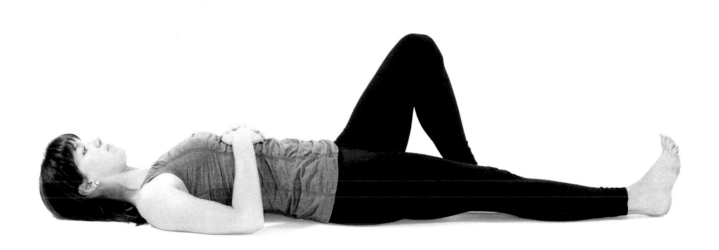

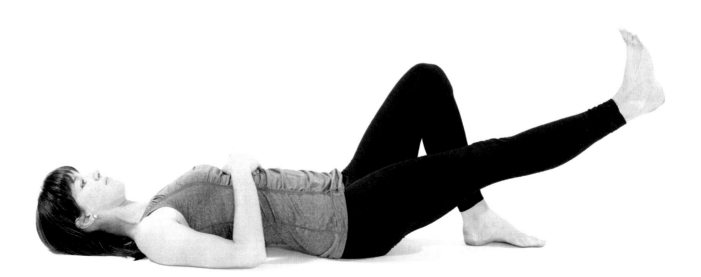

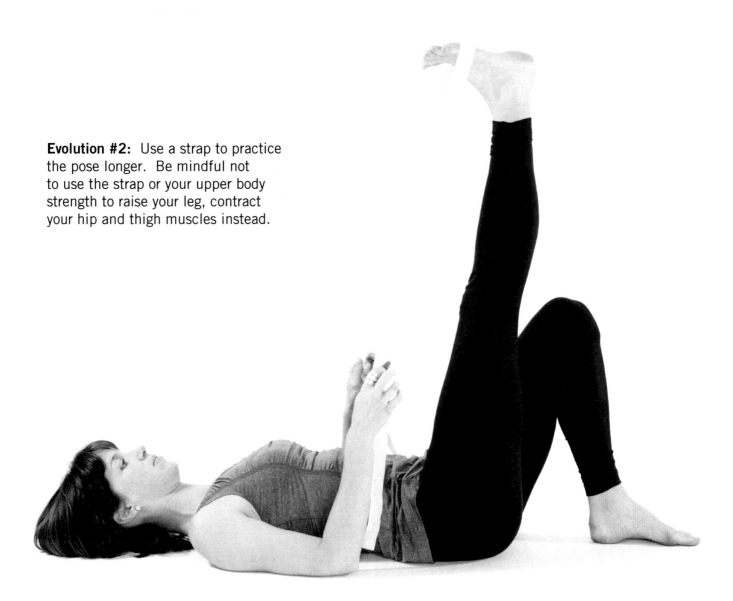

Evolution #2: Use a strap to practice the pose longer. Be mindful not to use the strap or your upper body strength to raise your leg, contract your hip and thigh muscles instead.

Bridge Pose - Setu Bandha Sarvangasana

Prop: Ball or block, and blanket (optional)

Prop Tip: When I talk about using a ball here, I am referring to a very light, inflatable ball. The ball should be roughly 9 inch in diameter and should give when you apply resistance to it.

How to: Lay on your back on the floor with your knees bent and your feet and knees hip width apart. If laying on your back bothers your spine, shoulders, or neck, place a thinly folded blanket under your shoulders and torso. Your neck and back of the head should be free of the support. Rest your arms next to you on the floor, elbows straight.

- Prep for the pose first. Engage your buttock muscles and deep lower abdominals before you lift to help stabilize the pelvis and spine.
- Press into the centre of your heels and slowly lift with ease.
- Hold for a few breaths, exhale as you lower back down. **Repeat for 4 breaths, gradually increasing the amount of time you hold the bridge.**

Tip: If bridge causes you back pain or strain, slowly release out of the pose. Adjust the distance of the feet from the body and work on the prep pose to master it.

Evolution: Ball/block

- Place a ball or a block between your inner thighs. Ensure the prop is the proper width to keep your knees and feet hip width apart.
- Gently squeeze the prop with your inner thighs. Be mindful not to tense in other areas of the body, only the inner thighs need work here.
- Inhale and lift as above. Continue to squeeze the prop to maintain your knee-hip alignment.

Tip: If the use of the prop causes you knee pain, lower down and readjust the amount of pressure you are applying into the prop before lifting again. If you can't avoid knee pain in this variation, change your prop or continue to practice bridge without a prop.

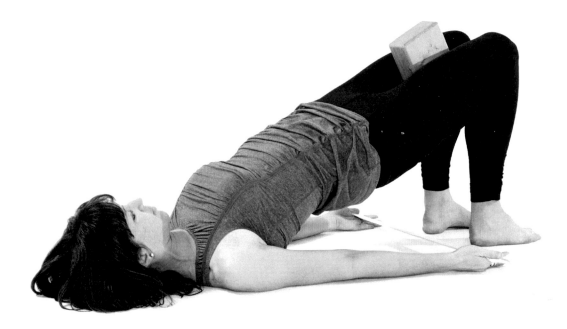

The Hips

Clamshell

Props (optional): Blanket or firm pillow for under the head

How to:

- Lay on your left side and support your head so that your neck is in a neutral position either with your arm, a blanket, or a firm pillow.
- Bend your hips and knees, then lean forward slightly.
- Keep your feet together as you inhale and lift your top leg, exhale to lower with control. **Repeat for 10 breaths moving with the breath then switch sides**.

Tip: Place your top hand on your top pelvic bone. With your fingers, feel for any involvement of the muscles that cross the front of the hip - you want none! Lift only as high as you need to without these muscles kicking in to ensure you work the correct muscle of the hip we want to use.

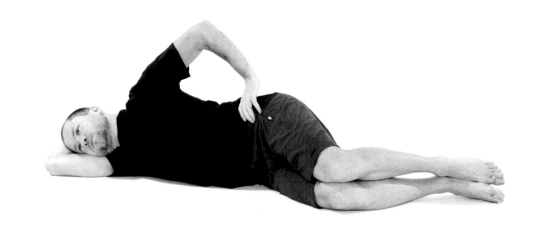

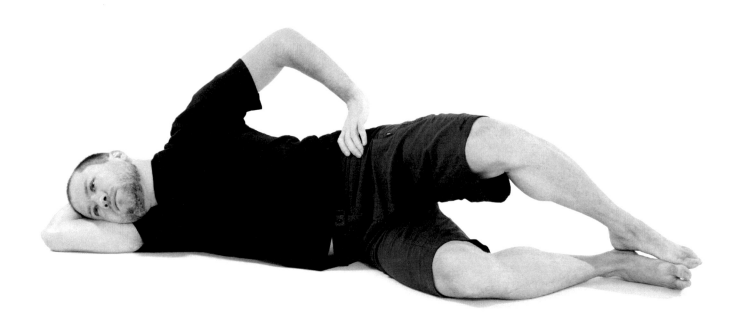

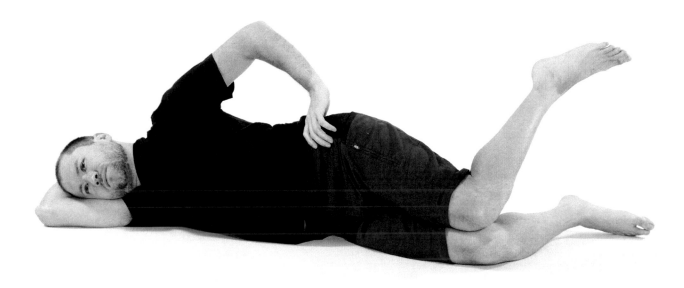

Reverse Clamshell

Props (optional): Blanket or firm pillow for under the head

How to:

- Lay just as you did for clamshells except with your knees back in line with your hips.
- Keep your knees together as you inhale and internally rotate your top thigh bone in the hip socket; your foot will lift as a result. Exhale as you rotate your thigh back to neutral with control.
- **Repeat for 10 breaths, moving with the breath then switch sides.**

Tip: The point here is not to lift your foot higher. Rather, you want to improve the range of motion of the thigh bone in the hip socket.

Evolution: Elevated Clamshell & Reverse Clamshell

Perform this more advanced variation of both the clamshell and reverse clamshell once you have mastered the above to continue to improve your strength and coordination.

How to:

- Start with your top leg lifted so your knee is lined up with your hip.
- Pivot around your foot (for lifted clamshells) or around your knee (for lifted reverse clamshells)

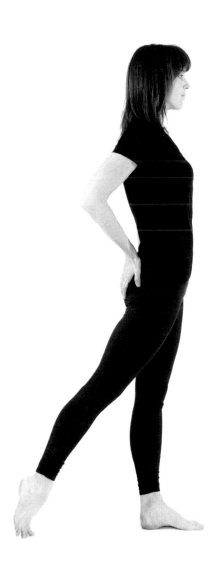

Standing Hip Extensions - Natarajasana Prep

Props (optional): Table, chair or wall

Preparation:

- Stand next to a support for balance.
- Step your right foot back a couple of inches, keep your knee slightly bent.
- Prep for the hip extension by engaging your right buttock muscle without rotating the leg.
- Hold for a breath, then release. **Repeat for 10 breaths then switch legs**.
- Work on the preparation for as long as you need to feel the buttock muscle engagement before moving on to the full hip extension. The same goes if you have to compensate by arching the back or involving your lower back or hamstring (back of the thigh) muscles.

Tip: The point here is not to lift your foot. Rather, you want to improve the range of motion of your thigh bone in the hip socket.

Hip Extension:

- Start as you did for the preparation.
- Engage your deep lower abdominals to help support the pelvis and spine in a neutral position.
- Inhale and pull your right leg back using the buttock muscles.
- Hold for a breath, then exhale to lower the leg.
- **Repeat for 10 breaths, moving with the breath, then switch legs**.

Prone Hip Extensions - Salabasana Prep

Props: Blankets

How to: Lay on your stomach, on the floor. Fold your arms in front of you and place your forehead on your forearms to keep your neck in a neutral position. Use a support like a folded blanket under your forehead as needed. The same goes for your lower back; if your pelvis has a tendency to tilt forward so that you end up with an exaggerated curve in your low back, place a second folded blanket under your belly and pelvic bones.

Preparation: As in Natarajasana

Straight Leg:

- Start with your legs hip-width apart.
- Take your right foot to the edge of your mat. If you aren't using a mat, estimate another inch out to the side.
- Inhale and lift the right leg from the buttock, exhale to release.
- **Repeat 10x, switch to the left leg**.

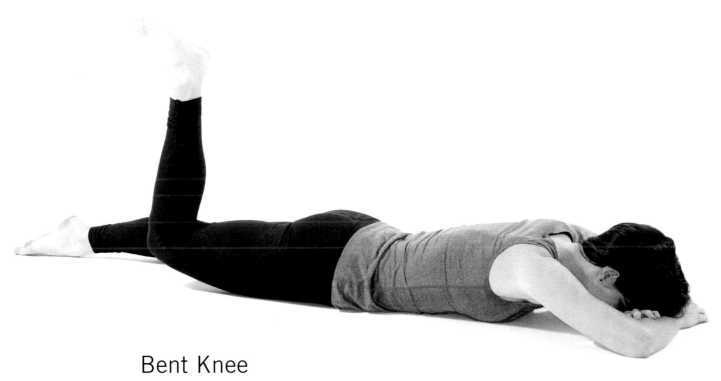

Bent Knee

- Start the same why as in the straight-leg version.
- Bend your right knee to 90°.
- Inhale and lift the right leg from the buttock without changing the angle of the knee. Exhale to release.
- **Repeat for 10 breaths then switch legs.**

Tip: In both variations, if your lower back is speaking to you in any way, you are lifting your leg too high. Only lift your leg to a height where you feel no lower back pain, no bracing of your lower back muscles, and no movement of your pelvis.

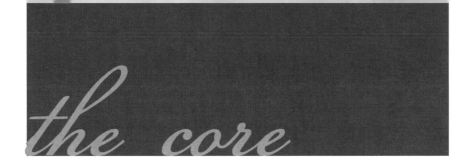

the core

The Girdle: Abdominal Contraction

How-to: Lay on your back, on the floor, knees bent with feet and knees hip width apart. Place your hands on your pelvic bones, those bony parts on either side of the front of your pelvis. With your fingers, feel for a gentle contraction of your deeper abdominal muscles; avoid gripping or holding your breath. Your spine should stay neutral so your low back maintains its natural curve and avoids flattening to the floor.

Tip: If you aren't sure where neutral spine is, tilt your pelvis forward and back without forcing to get a sense of your range. Settle in the middle to find neutral spine.

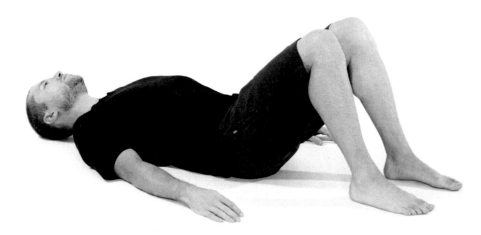

Butterfly: Knee Drops

Bonus: This sequence is wonderful for teaching core coordination and stabilization of the pelvis and spine.

How to: Start as in 'The Girdle' above. From there, add single leg alternating and double leg knee drops or butterflies.

Single Leg Alternating

- Inhale and lower your right leg out to the floor, exhale to pull it back up.
- Alternate with the left leg.
- Keep your pelvis still as you move and be careful not to rock towards the leg you are lowering.
- **Repeat for 10 breaths per leg**.

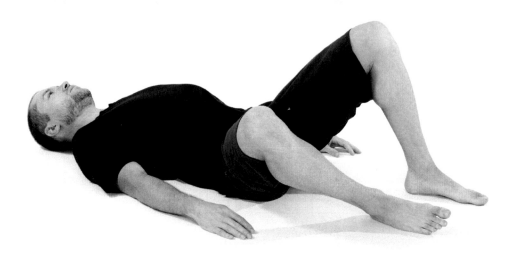

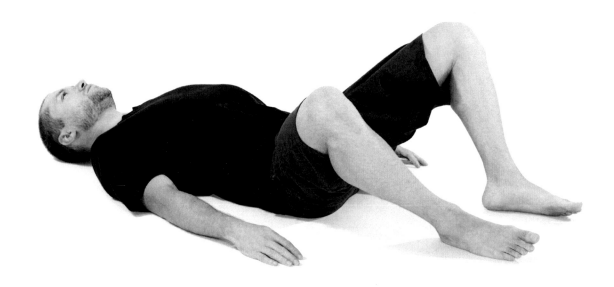

Double Leg

- Inhale and lower both legs to the floor
- Keep your pelvis still throughout and be careful not to tilt to either side
- Exhale while pulling your legs back up.
- **Repeat for 10 breaths**.

Cat Pose - Marjaryasana

Props: A folded or rolled mat or a blanket (optional, for the kneeling variation), or chair (for the seated variation)

How to: First decide which version is right for you. This will help you decide which props to use. For example, if you have arthritis in your wrists, knees or ankles, opt for the seated option.

Even those with healthy knees and ankles may find the kneeling version hard on their joints. Use a folded mat or blanket under the palms of the hands and another folded mat or blanket under the knees and shins. We want to add padding for the joints without drastically changing the alignment of the pose. Your wrists and knees should stay at the same height.

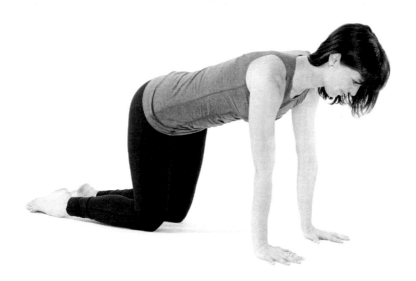

- Exhale as you round your mid back. Think of drawing your back ribs up as you contract the muscles of your abdomen.
- Inhale to lift the sternum, draw your shoulder blades into your back, and contract the muscles of your mid-back.
- Let your lower back and neck move as an extension of the mid-back.
- **Repeat for 10 breaths** as you move with the breath.

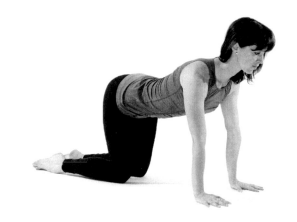

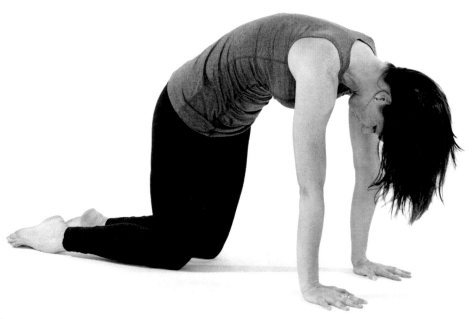

Variation: Seated Cat Pose

How to: Sit on a chair, spine straight but away from the chair back. Have your knees bent at 90 degrees and your feet flat on the floor; use a prop under the feet if needed. Breathe as with the kneeling version, **repeat for 10 breaths**.

You may also practice this pose seated cross legged as below.

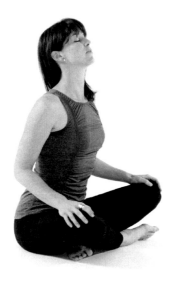 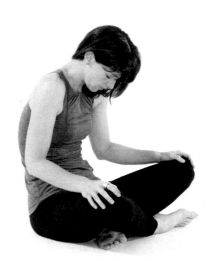

Downward-facing Hero - Adho Mukha Virasana

Prop: Blanket or edge of your bed

How to: Kneel on your hands and knees. As with Cat Pose, use folded blankets or a mat for additional support under your shins, knees, and wrists to reduce pressure on your joints. If you are practicing from the edge of a bed, let the front of your ankles rest on the edge while your feet dangle off.

Classic Pose

- Keep your big toes together while you move your knees wider than hip width apart.
- Bring your pelvis to neutral. If you do not know where neutral is, tilt your pelvis all the way forward then all the way back and settle in the middle.
- As you keep your pelvis still, exhale and start to slowly pull your hips back without rounding your low back or sitting on your heels.
- If you feel any discomfort through the front of your hips, take your knees wider.
- **Hold for several breaths, inhale to pull yourself forward. Repeat for 6 breaths**.

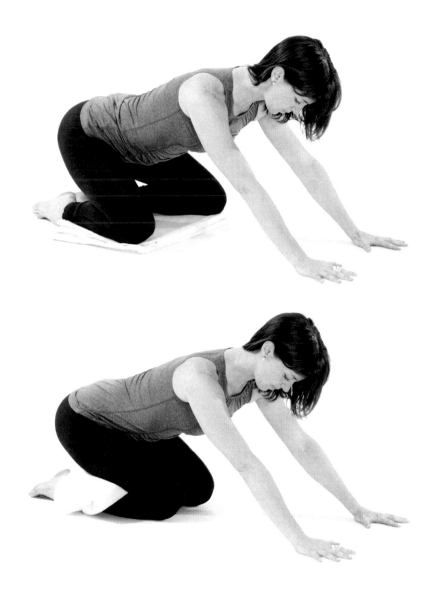

Narrow Advanced Version

How to: If your hips and back are happy in the classic version, practice Downward Facing Hero with your knees and feet hip distance apart.

Tip: The closer your knees and feet are to hip width, the more advanced the pose for the hips and lower back. **Keep your hips and knees happy by never taking your feet wider than hip width.**

Restorative Variation

Use additional props behind the knees, under the ankles and under the torso and forehead for a restorative version of the pose. Hold for a couple of minutes, inhale to bring yourself up.

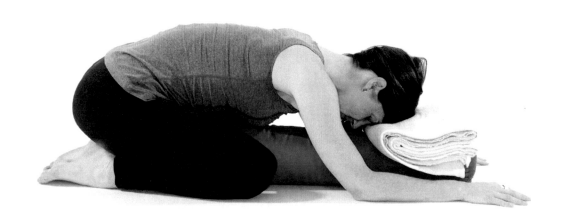

Evolution: The Spine - Plank Variation

Link: Start as in Cat Pose.

How to: Walk your knees back until you feel your lower abdominals engage.

- Keep your spine, pelvis and shoulders still.

- Hold for **5 breaths** then exhale to walk the knees back. **Repeat 4x.**

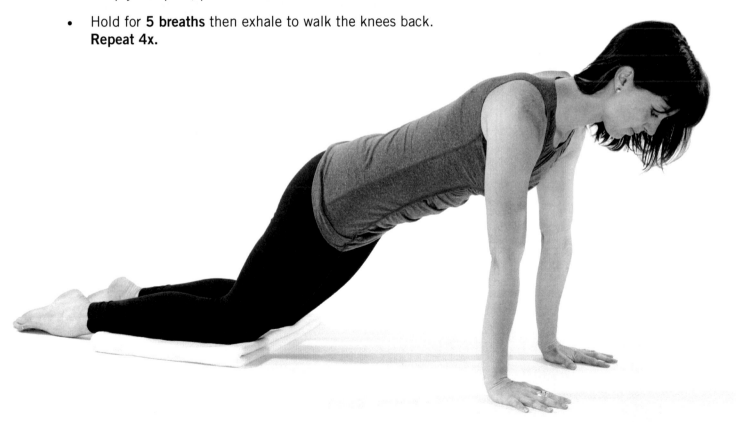

The Neck

Is your head on straight?

Posture Tip: My 3 finger Test

Here is an easy way to feel the curvature of your cervical spine, or your neck, and to discover how your noggin' is sitting on your spine.

How to: Get in touch with your inner Girl Scout and hold the middle three fingers on one hand together. Use your fingers to feel the back on your neck. If the back of your neck feels flat and hard, you have lost the natural curve of your cervical spine; if the curve feels extreme and your fingers are squeezed by your neck muscles, your neck is likely hyperextended with your head tipped backwards. Aim for something in the middle. Ideally, you should have a gentle curve in your neck.

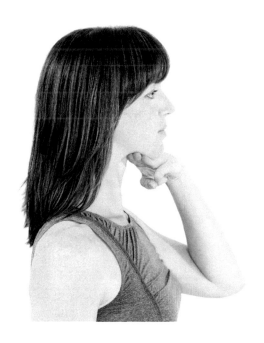

Use the same three fingers to feel under your chin. As a general rule, three fingers is the average distance you should have from the front of your throat to the tip of your chin. If the space is larger, this could mean you have a tendency towards a forward head position.

Be aware of your tendency where the above two posture checks are concerned. If you can't adjust either the curvature of your neck or the position of the head without it feeling forced, then work through the following upper body sequence. This will help you gradually improve function and mobility in your cervical spine, improve your posture, and ultimately the health of your neck joints.

4 T's: Turn, Tilt, Tuck, and Tip

How to: Here we explore the range of motion of your neck. Start in a seated or standing position with your back straight and your gaze forward. Perform the '3 Finger Test' first to help you begin from a neutral head position.

Golden Rules: With each "T", move with ease, control, and stop before you feel strain or a stretch sensation on the opposite side of your neck.

1. **Turn**: Exhale and turn your head gently to the right. Inhale to return to centre. Repeat to the other side. **Repeat for 4 breaths**.

2. **Tilt**: Exhale and tilt your head gently to the right. Inhale to pull your head back up. Repeat to the other side. **Repeat for 4 breaths**.

3. **Tuck**: Exhale and contract the muscles along the front of your neck to tuck your chin to your chest. Keep the rest of your spine straight. Move your chin to your right shoulder as you keep your chin tucked. Return to centre and then move slowly to the left. Return to center and inhale to pull your head back up. **Repeat for 4 breaths**.

4. Inhale as you tip your chin up and back. Pull your head back using the muscles along the back of your neck but without losing control or straining the front of the neck. Exhale to pull your head back to center. **Repeat for 4 breaths**.

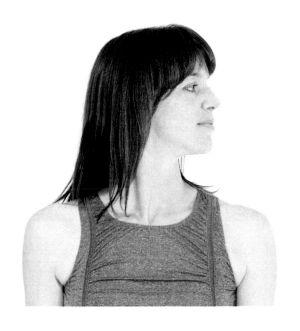

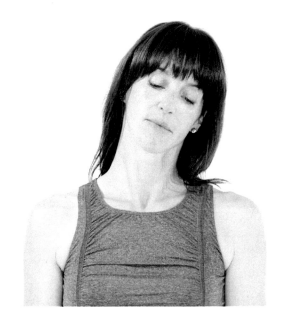

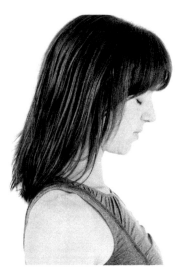

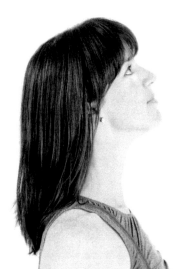

Bonus Ninja Move: Circles

Get your groove back and move to your own beat with this variation of the neck range of motion. Make circles with your neck. Start with small circles first then increase the size as your range improves. **Perform for 4 breaths in a clockwise direction then do 4 breaths counterclockwise.**

Swimmer's Roll

How to: Get in touch with your inner swimmer. Start with your right shoulder. Roll your shoulder up, back, and down to make a circle and create a flowing movement. **Alternate shoulders for 10 breaths.**

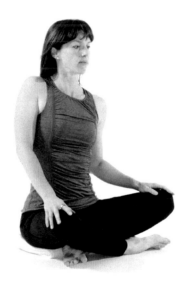

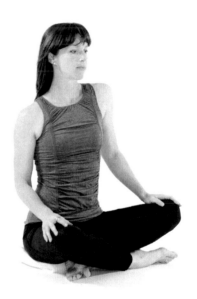

Variation: Single Shoulder Roll

Start with your right shoulder creating small circles and gradually progressing to larger ones. **Repeat for 10 breaths, switch shoulders**.

Variation: Double Shoulder Roll

Roll both shoulders together. **Repeat for 10 breaths**.

Side Shoulder Slide

Prop: Folded blanket or pillow

How to: Lay on your right side. Use a folded blanket, block, or your arm if your shoulder is healthy to support your head. Lean forward slightly and bend at your hips and knees. You should feel comfortable and relaxed, not off balance as if you were about to roll backwards.

- Inhale and roll your top (left) shoulder back.
- Draw your left shoulder blade down the back as if you were trying to place it in your back pant pocket; gently squeeze without pinching your shoulder blade towards your spine.
- Exhale to release. **Repeat for 6 breaths, then switch sides**.

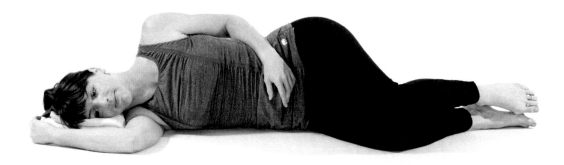

Evolution: Add the hip

At the same time as you do the shoulder slide, draw the outer left hip up towards the rib cage. Squeeze for a breath, exhale to release. **Repeat for 10 breaths**.

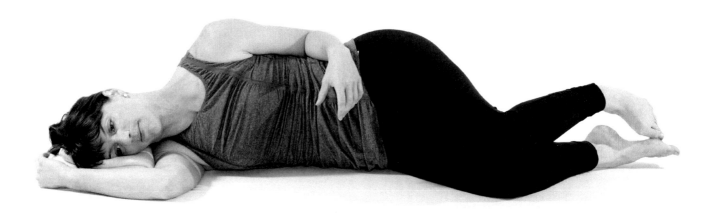

Eagle Arms - Garudasana

Prep:

- Lift your right arm up in front of you and bend your elbow to 90 degrees, palm in.
- Take your left hand and hold the outside of your right elbow. Inhale and gently press your right elbow into your hand as you engage your upper outer back muscles; exhale to release.
- Be mindful not to press back with your left hand! Use it as resistance only.
- Repeat for 3 breaths.
- **Switch to hold the inner elbow**. Contract your chest muscles as you gently press in, exhale to release. **Repeat for 3 breaths**.
- **Repeat the entire prep with the other arm.**

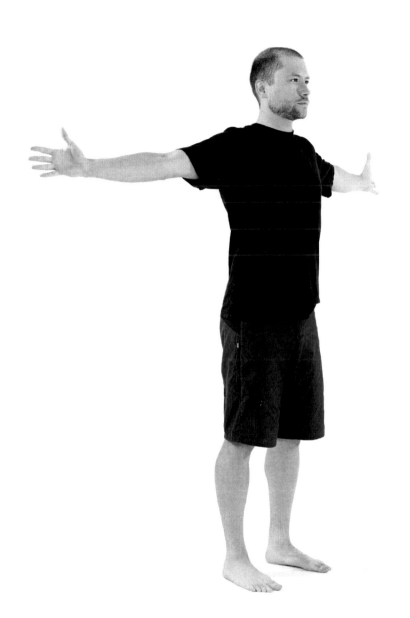

Hug Approach - Arm Reach

How to:

- Roll your shoulders back so your arms rotate and your palms face forward.
- Inhale and lift your arms out to the sides to shoulder height.
- Fan your hands, spread your fingers, and breathe.
- Reach back without pinching the shoulder blades together.
- Your shoulders should remain down away from your ears
- **Hold for 4 breaths, exhale as you lower the arms. Repeat 4x.**

Give Yourself a Hug

How to: Lift your arms as you did for the 'Hug Approach - Arm Reach'

- Exhale as you engage your chest. Pull your arms in and cross your right arm over left.
- Reach around your shoulders and give yourself a hug.
- Gently squeeze your chest muscles. **Hold for 6 breaths, inhale to open your arms.**
- Repeat by crossing your arms the other way.

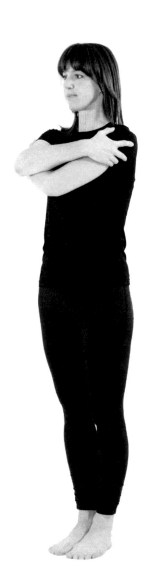

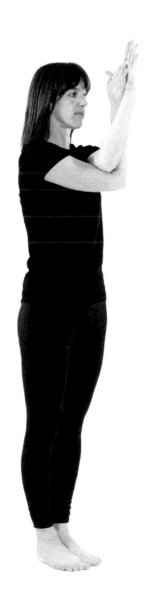

Full Pose

- Lift both arms up in front of you, bend your elbows to 90 degrees palms in.
- Now cross your left arm over your right as shown and engage your chest muscles.
- Depending on your flexibility and mobility, you may be able to cross anywhere from your wrists to your elbows. Whatever the case, your shoulders should remain down away from your ears.
- **Hold for 6 breaths, switch the cross.**

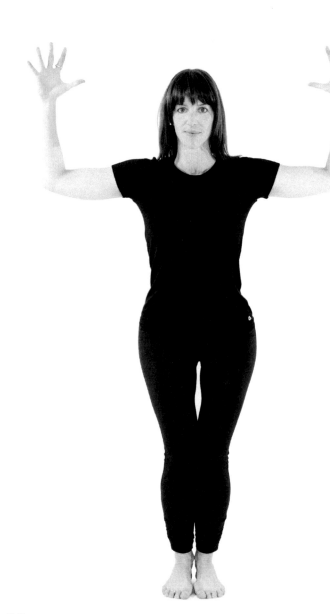

Synchro Arms - Biceps/Triceps

How to: Lift your arms as you did for the 'Arm Reach'. Bend your elbows and come into cactus pose with your palms forward and elbows at 90 degrees. Keep the shoulders down away from your ears.

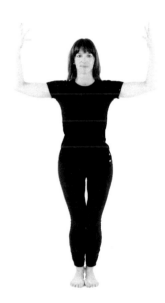

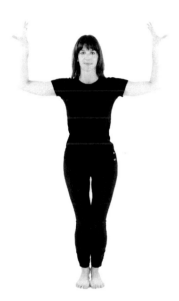

- Inhale and rotate your upper arms to draw your inner elbows towards your armpits. Feel your biceps contract.

- Exhale and rotate your upper arms as to bring your outer elbows closer to the back of your armpits. Feel your triceps contract.
- **Alternate 10x in each direction, exhale to bring your arms down.**

Chest Release on a Folded Blanket

Props: Folded blanket (eg. a thick Mexican or Indian blanket)

Prop tip: If you don't have the ideal blanket, a pool noodle or rolled mat with a block are good alternatives.

How to: Fold your blanket so it is long enough to support your entire spine from head to tailbone. Fold it in such a way that it is no wider than 6 inches, or narrower than the width of your back. Remove any creases, lumps, or bumps from the folds to ensure optimal comfort when you eventually lay along it.

- Lay sideways next to the blanket and roll onto it.
- Make sure everything from your head to your buttocks is supported.
- Bend your knees and place your feet on the floor on either side of the blanket.
- Roll your arms to the floor and turn your arms so your palms face up.
- This might be enough for you to open the chest and broaden the collarbones in a way that feels comfortable.

Evolution:

- Slide the arms along the floor so the arms form a 'V'.
- Continue until your hands are in line with the shoulders to create a 'T'
- Bend the elbows to 45 degrees, gradually moving to 90 degrees.

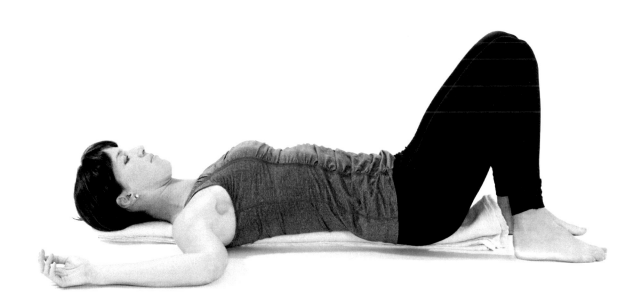

Use Your Hands and Wrists to Their Full Potential

Our lifestyle, activities, and health often determine how we use and misuse our hands. If you spend most of your time typing, writing and texting, you are doing an injustice to your hands. If you jump into yoga poses before your wrists are ready, you are not going to like it.   Having said that, if you shy away from certain movements because of arthritis pain in your fingers and wrists, you are doing your joints a disservice. You don't have to flail around to feel the benefits but you do have to get your hands movin' and groovin'.

Here are some mini yoga moves you can practice daily to help improve mobility and strength plus eliminate pain in your hands, wrists and fingers. Avoid forcing the movements but rather breathe normally, move slowly, and don't do any move that causes your pain to increase.

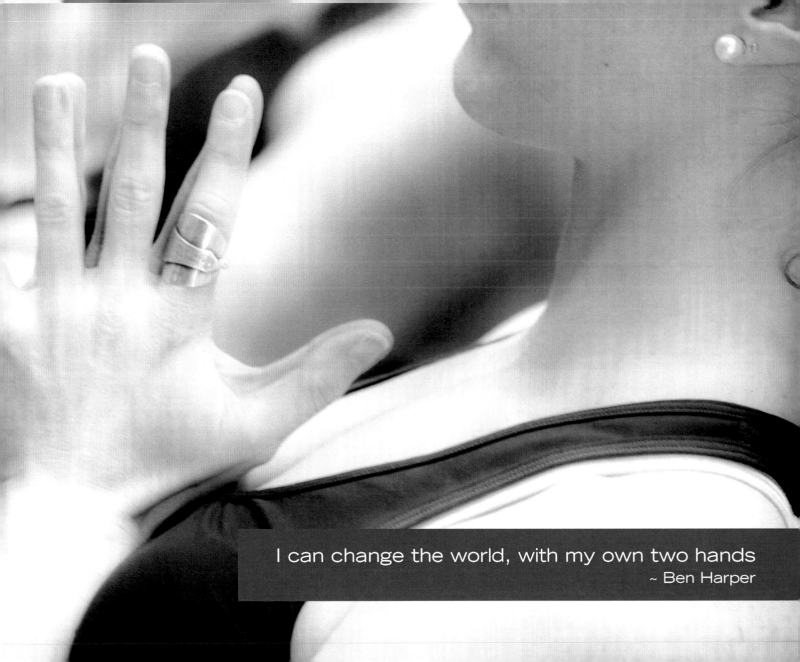

I can change the world, with my own two hands
~ Ben Harper

Adho Mukha Svanasana - Hands Only

Props: A flat surface like a desk, table, or counter top.

Adho Mukha Svananasana, or Downward Facing Dog as it is more commonly known, is one of the most recognizable yoga poses. The grounding of the hands in this pose is an important cue students often hear from their teachers.

Arthritis in the hands and wrists along with poor flexibility and mobility in the shoulders make this pose inaccessible to many. Here we introduce a new take on the traditional yoga pose that requires none of the weight bearing or shoulder flexibility but offers every bit of the benefit of a fanned hand position. Consider it Downward Dog without the down.

- Place your hands palms down on a flat surface and gently spread your fingers.
- Reach your fingers away as if you were trying to lengthen them out.
- Gently ground evenly into all the points of your hands. Do not force your hand down but rather focus on having all points of the hands touching the surface.
- Pay special attention to grounding into areas of your hands that lift, e.g., the space between your thumb and index finger and your inner palm are sneaky areas that often lift.
- Notice if you are tensing in any part of the neck or face. Relax and breathe normally.
- **Hold for 4 breaths**.

Relax and repeat 4 times

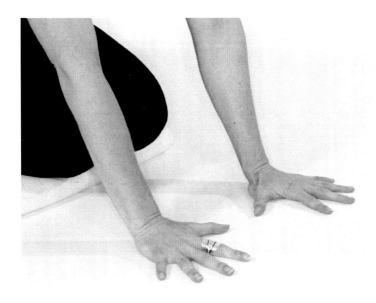

Tip**Tip**: Use a mirrored or glass surface or a mat to ground into. When you take your hands away you will see where you were applying pressure.

The Piano Player

You don't need to take piano lessons to master this move.

How to: Start as in Adho Mukha Svanasana above. Lift your thumbs and then place them back down. Continue along the hand as you lift each finger in succession without lifting the palm off the table. Move slowly and with ease. Once you reach your pinky, reverse the sequence. **Repeat 5x both directions then switch hands**.

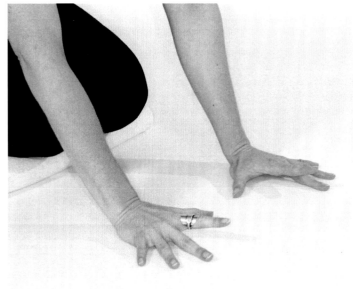

73

Namaste/Anjali Mudra

How to:

- Bring your hands to chest height, press your palms together and fan your fingers out.
- Tilt your hands out slightly so the base of your thumbs rest at your sternum.
- Gently press the points of your hands together. Be mindful to keep even pressure in your hands, one hand should not dominate the other.
- Your hands should work together and be friends here!
- **Hold for 4 breaths, repeat 5x.**

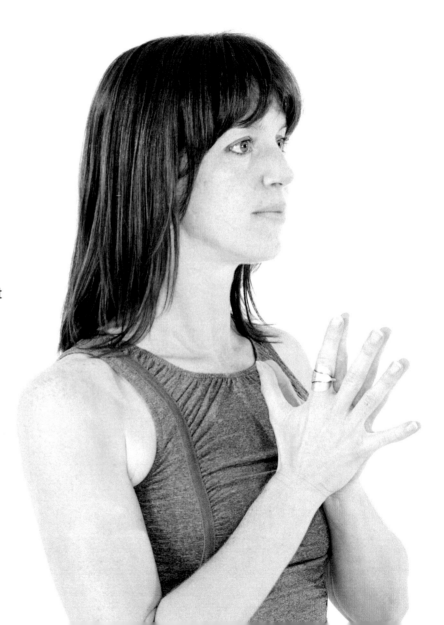

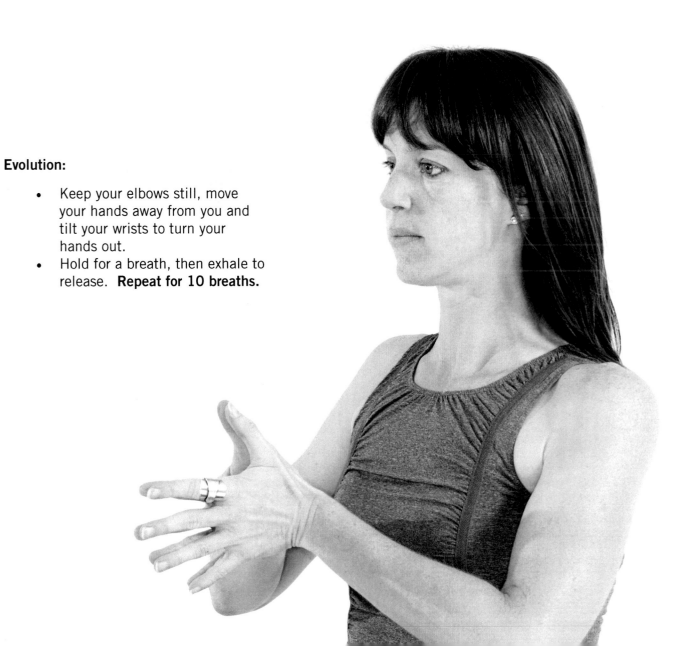

Evolution:

- Keep your elbows still, move your hands away from you and tilt your wrists to turn your hands out.
- Hold for a breath, then exhale to release. **Repeat for 10 breaths.**

The Surfer and The Server: Forearm Rotation

How to: Stand or sit with your arms at your sides, and palms facing down. Keep your shoulders quiet as you rotate your upper arms back. Keep your upper arms still as you rotate your forearms so the palms face down. **Rotate back and forth for 10 breaths.**

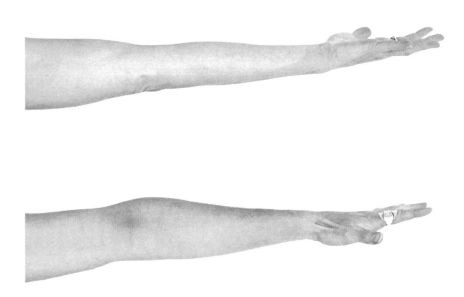

Interlocked Hands - Parvatasana

How to: Lift your arms to shoulder height. Keep your shoulders down away from your ears. Interlock your fingers, touch your thumbs and gently straighten your arms. **Hold for 6 breaths then exhale to release the arms.**

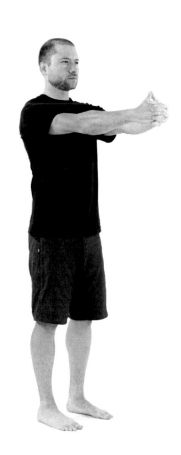

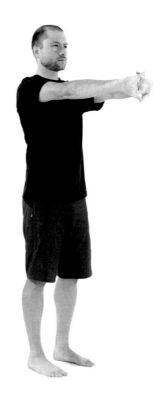

Evolution: Turn your arms so your palms face out.

Full Pose: Start as above. Inhale as you lift your arms overhead and keep your shoulders down. If you have to bend your elbows or arch your back to lift your arms, you have gone too far. Whatever your range, **hold the pose for 6 breaths as you open the palms and lengthen the arms**.

Tip: Avoid hyperextending your elbows by engaging your biceps. If you are not sure if you are hyperextending, keep a small bend in your elbows.

Hand Mudras

Tip: Hand Mudras can be done seated or standing. If touching your thumbs and fingers together is difficult, not to worry. The point is to work your thumbs and fingers closer each time. Do what you can, every move has a benefit.

How to:

- Sit crosslegged or in a chair.
- Place the back of your hands comfortably on your thighs or knees
- Start with your index finger, touch the tip of your finger to the tip of your thumb.
- Work along your hand until you get to your pinky, then start back towards your index finger.
- **Repeat 5 times in both directions for each hand**.

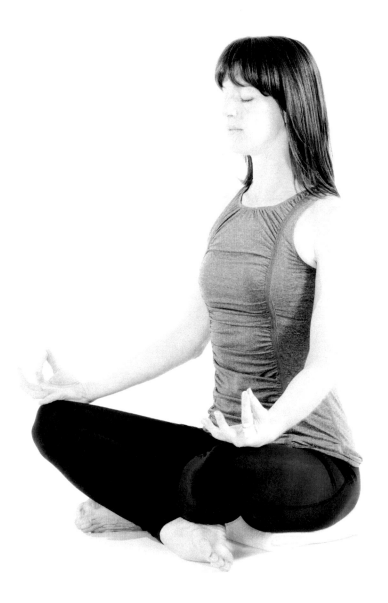

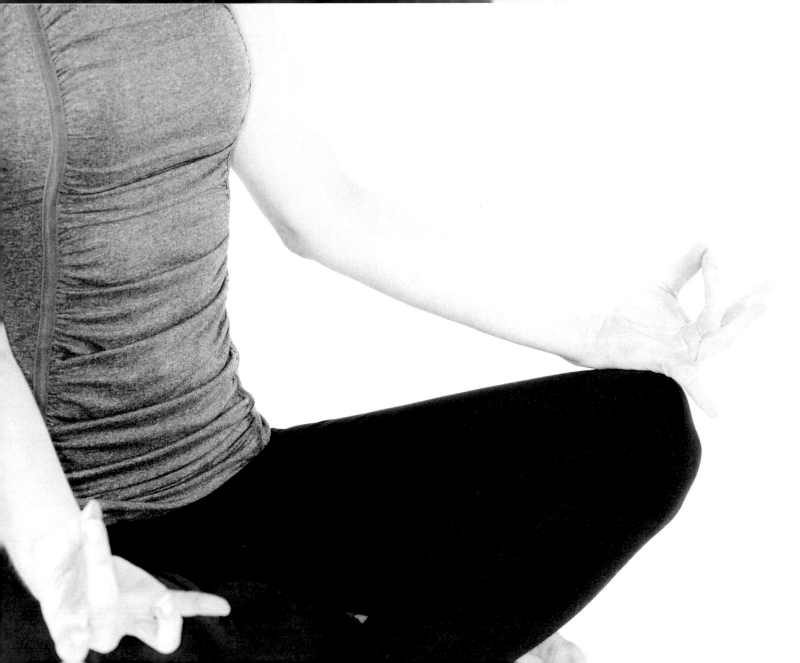

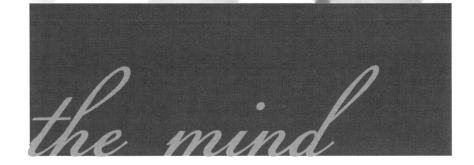

the mind

I will let you in on a little secret: if your psychological bucket is empty it will be much harder to feel good physically. The opposite is also true: when your mental bucket is full, you will feel better physically and will be better able to manage stress and pain. The asanas or yoga poses are there to help you get rid of the physical roadblocks to create the space for mental wellbeing. But if we are drained emotionally how can we even make it to the mat?

Remember Rule #7.

Progress comes when you take care of ALL of you. The best way to do this: use your brain power. Believe you can feel better. If you are doing something that will help you improve your health, you will feel better. Trust in your ability to heal chances are, you will live a happier life.

If the above prospect sounds silly or esoteric, use the other limbs of yoga to help you get there, namely Pratyahara, Pranayama, Dharana, and Dhyana. Don't let the Sanskrit names fool you, these are real life yoga ninja skills. You want them on your side when battling insomnia, pain, stress, and depression.

Pratyahara

The best way I can explain the fifth limb of yoga is by using a comparison.   Pratyahara, or the practice of closing off your senses, is like creating your very own sensory deprivation tank. No sound, no light, and no sensation.

Savasana, the pose at the end of a yoga class that everyone loves so much, is priming you for a pratyahara practice. In Savasana we lay still, close our eyes, and turn off our ears. We relax deeply and become physically comfortable. When we are still our mind is allowed to be quiet. Before you know it, the sensory noise that usually has a hold on you losses its grip. The mental noise and internal dialogue might still be there but you are no longer being distracted by it. Those voices in your head? Gone.

Breath Awareness: Pranayama

> When you arise in the morning
> Think of what a precious privilege it is to be alive
> To breathe, to think, to enjoy, to love.
> ~ Marcus Aurelius

Pranayama translates to "elongation of energy" and by controlling our breathing we can learn to control our energy. Translation: relax and manage our stress.

B.K.S. Iyengar teaches us that our practice can backfire on us if we dive into pranayama without first having mastered our asana skills. So what is a yoga ninja to do? Start with the basics.

Take a deep breath. Exhale. Here we go.

Breath Awareness

The first plan of attack when practicing breath awareness is to, wait for it, breathe.

The next plan of attack is to decide how to get comfortable. Sit or lay down? Choose a pose that will give you the most success. If you do not think you can sit for a decent period of time, start in a reclined position. To be an adept ninja however, you must practice both. By exploring your breath in both a seated and a reclined position you can fully experience the difference in the mechanics of how you breathe in each.

Tip: When you first start your practice, you will feel uncomfortable. Figure out if the discomfort comes from a real need to move and adjust or if it comes from that pesky voice in your head trying to get in the way.

The main difference in how you breathe is that when you lay down, your rib cage stays relatively still; in a seated position there is a natural movement of the ribs. Once you feel and recognize the difference between the two, your movements in your yoga poses will become easier.

The last consideration is to leave your ego at the door. We are practicing giving up control which can be hard for some of us. Enjoy the journey and the excuse to let things happen as they may. No judgements, no analysis, only acceptance.

Seated Breathing

Movement of the ribs

In an upright position there are two main movements of the rib cage. During a very deep breath, the sternum moves forward and lifts.

Tip: To feel this in your own body, open your mouth slightly and take in a few deep breaths.

The other movement of the rib cage is less obvious. During normal breathing, the upper chest becomes quiet and movement is more noticeable in the lower ribs. The lower ribs expand out in all directions, but especially out.

Tip: Feel the movement by placing your hands on the sides of your ribcage.

Practice:

1. Sit tall in a seated position on the floor or in a chair. Gently lift your spine so that the rib cage, the abdomen, and the back are free to move.

2. Rest your hands on your thighs. Close your eyes and turn your attention to your breathing. Notice the rhythm, the depth, and the ease of your exhalations and inhalations.

3. Let the muscles of your abdomen and back support your spine without straining. Let the muscles of your ribcage relax to allow more space to breathe.

4. Notice how your rib cage expands out, forward, and back.

5. Recognize the normal movement created by the diaphragm in a seated pose. This is the first step to mastering breath awareness which will help you to improve your concentration and relax your breathing style. The result: less temptation to control your breath.

6. Practice for a couple of minutes.

Prone Breathing - On Your Stomach

Movement of the back

You get to lay on your tummy for this one. If the floor isn't accessible to you, a bed will do nicely.

Tip: Keep your low back happy by adding extra support under the pelvis, and lower belly in the form of a thinly folded blanket.

Tip: Unless you are lucky enough to have your own massage table with a head rest, your head should rest on your arms or be turned to the side. For the latter, rest on your ear, cheek or somewhere in between at a range that feels comfortable and easy. If this is awkward or painful, add a thin blanket under the head.

Practice:

1. Lay on your stomach, let your back expand with each inhalation. Notice the change in the way your breath between this position and the previous seated pose.

2. Allow your shoulders to comfortably roll forward towards to the floor. Your palms will face up with the thumbs pointing in towards your body.

3. Breathe into your back ribs. Let the middle of your back and back of the ribcage rise and fall with the rhythm of your breath. Enjoy the feeling of lift that is created as you inhale.

4. Feel the space between your shoulder blades move; visualize the area lifting and expanding with each inhalation.

5. Enjoy the exploration of prone breathing for a couple of minutes.

Supine Breathing - On Your Back

When you lay on your back, your belly rises with the inhalation and falls with the exhalation with the movement of the diaphram.

Tip: Feel the movement by placing your hands on your lower ribs.

Tip: To keep your lower back happy, add a bolster, pillow, folded blanket, or rolled mat under your knees for support. You can add a thinly folded blanket under your head too for added coziness.

Practice:

1. Lie on your back. Roll your shoulders down to the floor and relax your upper arms; your palms will face up and your thumbs out.

2. Bring your awareness to your breath and enjoy the rhythm made by your exhalations and inhalations. Let your breathing happen naturally without trying to control or force it.

3. With your hands on your low ribs, feel your hands pull apart gently as your abdomen lifts with the inhalation. You hands will draw back together as your low ribs fall naturally with the exhalation.

4. Give up control, observe, and experience each breath as it flows naturally into the next.

5. Watch your breath for a few minutes; let your body and mind unwind.

Evolution: If you can bring your arms to the floor over your head with ease, try this variation. Use another blanket under the arms for added support.